Metabolism Plan

The Ultimate Beginner's Metabolism Plan Diet Guide to Restore Your Energy, Detox & Cleanse Your Body, Lose Weight and Burn Body Fat Fast

By *Freddie Masterson*

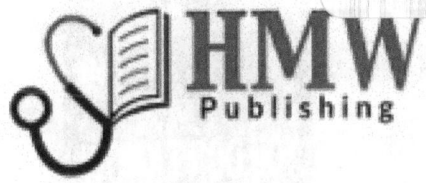

For more great books visit:

HMWPublishing.com

Get another book for Free

I want to thank you for purchasing this book and offer you another book (just as long and valuable as this book), "Health & Fitness Mistakes You Don't Know You're Making", completely free.

Visit the link below to signup and receive it:

www.hmwpublishing.com/gift

In this book, I will break down the most common health & fitness mistakes, you are probably committing right now, and I will reveal how you can easily get in the best shape of your life!

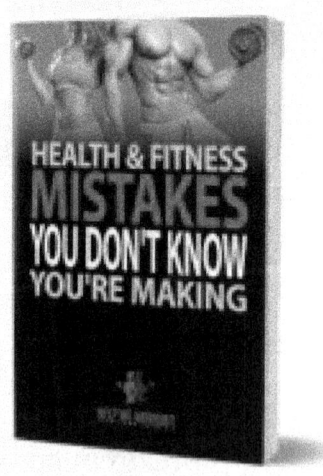

In addition to this valuable gift, you will also have an opportunity to get our new books for free, enter giveaways, and receive other valuable emails from me. Again, visit the link to sign up:

www.hmwpublishing.com/gift

TABLE OF CONTENTS

Introduction 2

Chapter 1: Let's Start With Some Basics 4

What is the Metabolism Plan? 7
Debunking some misconceptions about metabolism 9
Understanding How Metabolism Works 10
Why This Plan Works and Diets Don't! 11

Chapter 2: Ways To Lose Weight Without disturbing Your Personal Life Or Happiness distressing 13

Step 1 – Time Yourself (have a time plan) When Eating Meals by Placing a Timer 13
Step 2 – Tell Someone Who's Close to You That You Are Watching What You Eat 14
Step 3 – Create A Massive Batch of Green Tea and Freeze It 14
Step 4- If You Mess Up and Fall Off the Wagon, Get Back On 15
Step 5: Turn Off Your Phone, Tablet, And All Artificial Lights 2 Hours Before Bed. 15

Chapter 3: Key Commandments To Unlock Your Perfect Metabolism 17

Fix Your Sugar 17
The Importance of Fats 18
Heal Your Gut 18
Food Intolerances 20
Losing the Harmful Weight 20

Lowering Inflammation 22

Poor Sleep, Stress and A Life Spent On a Tablet or Phone 22

The Importance of Nutrients 23

Water, Water, Water 23

Brush Your Teeth After Meals! 24

Exercising More Efficiently................................24

Chapter 4: Simple Detox Guides 26

Importance of Detoxification...............................26

How to tell if my body needs to Detox? 26

Guide and Charts to Help You Detox the Right Way 28

Making it personal..28

Chapter 5: Eat And Cleanse At The Same Time. 32

Importance of incorporating the right foods into your plan..32

Delicious & Healthy fat-burning meals 32

When to eat to intensify detoxification?.............33

Chapter 6: 10 Minutes' Alternative Workout. Two Weeks Plan And What To Eat. 35

What Should Your Shopping List Look?............35

10-Minute Fat Burning Exercises Plan and 2-Weeks Diet Plan..35

Side-Plank Squat-Thrust Push-Up....................37

Squat-Thrust Push-Up with Leg Lifts...............38

Squat-Thrust Push-Up with Mountain Climbers 38

Here Are a Few Tips to Burn Fat While Toning and Defining Your Abs and Core 39

Equipment You Need: Yoga mat and A Record Timer 40

Challenge: Performing the Fat Burning Workout while doing the metabolism plan 40

Why is it okay to start with 10-minute workouts? 41

Doable 41

Gets you committed to the goal 41

These workouts are just as effective 42

Improved consistency 42

Chapter 7: How Will I Know If Things Are Working? 44

What Should You Expect? 44

Truth About Detoxing 44

Chapter 8: How Your Body Answers, What Does It Want, What Should You Do, Regularly 46

Tips for Long-Term Weight Loss Success 46

Here's Some Go- Tips for Long-Term Weight Loss 49

Broaden your taste buds. 49

Never go shopping on an empty stomach. 49

Taking this idea to another level is not going to a supermarket at all 50

How Often Should I Detox? 50

Do I Need to Give Up My Favourite Food, Alcohol, Coffee, Fast Foods? 52

Will I Lose Weight During the Detox? 55

Challenges to Expect-If Any.................................55
    Feeling sluggish..55
    Skin changes...56
    Mood changes 56

Chapter 9: Stable Metabolism Through Alternative Great/Easy/Fun Life Aspects......58

    Enjoyable Ways to Boost Metabolism in Achieving Homeostasis On Body Weight Regulation....58

    Dimming lights and wearing an earmark........58

    Setting your daily targets...............................59

    Doing exercise whenever you can....................60

Bonus Chapter: 30-Day Metabolism Meal Plan Tips!..61

    Let's Take a Look at The Typical 7 Day Meal Plan For Metabolism Diet: 62

    Breakfast 62

    Lunch..67

    Dinner 76

Conclusion 82

Final Words 85

About the Co-Author 86

INTRODUCTION

I want to thank you and congratulate you for purchasing the *"Metabolism Plan Diet"* book. This book contains proven steps and strategies on how you can lose weight and become healthier without having to go on a real diet. You will also discover how you can eat filling and delicious meals. Moreover, you will all learn the advantages of packing your food with veggies, fruits, nuts, legumes, and more. Likewise, you will also learn some helpful tips on how you can succeed in adopting the Metabolism Action Plan. Lastly, we even provide you with a sample meal plan and Metabolism action plan, which you can get started with right away!

Thanks again for purchasing this book, I hope you enjoy it!

Also, before you get started, I recommend you **joining our email newsletter** to receive updates on any upcoming new book releases or promotions. You can sign-up for free, and as a bonus, you will receive a free gift. Our *"Health & Fitness Mistakes You Don't Know You're Making"* book! This book has been written to demystify, expose the top do's and don'ts and to finally equip you with the information you need to get in the best shape of your life. Due to the overwhelming amount of mis-information and lies told by magazines and self-proclaimed "gurus", it's becoming harder and harder to get reliable information to get in shape. As opposed to having to go through dozens of biased, unreliable and un-trustworthy sources to get your health & fitness information. Everything you need to help you has been broken down in this book for you to easily follow and to immediately get results to achieve your desired fitness goals in the shortest amount of time.

Once again, to join our free email newsletter and to receive a free copy of this valuable book, please visit the link and signup now: www.hmwpublishing.com/gift

Chapter 1: Let's Start With Some Basics

Before reading further:

If this is something you are serious about, and the 30-day plan is the one you want to adhere to, then make a table. It should look pretty similar to this (you can use this one if you want). Print it out, save to Google drive and use it as we go forward:

	Day 1	Day 2	Day 3	Day 4	Day 5	Day 6	Day 7
Weight*							
Food Intake							
Bowel Movement?							
Hours of Sleep							
Approx. Calories							
Exercise							
General Feeling							
Psoriasis **							

*Do not weigh yourself daily. Weigh yourself at the start of the metabolism plan and then every five days. Pick a time, and stick to it each time you weigh yourself (sometime in the morning, preferably). Don't weigh yourself in the week preceding your period if you are a female.

To make the whole process a little more insightful, make a note of any autoimmune diseases that you might have; for example, candida. The idea here is to try and observe, how the diet affects symptoms of these disorders. Keeping track of everything will help you understand, how your body is reacting to the metabolism diet and the exercise changes. It also gives you a sense of control, since you are so involved in all the minute and drastic changes that take place during 30 days. The metabolism diet is so personal because you are the one who's calling the shots. You are the one in control. If for example, you are constipated; then you know that you need to add more fiber to your diet. Simultaneously also maintain the log any particular food that you think could be causing constipation. Repeat this process of recording and altering the menu as you move further towards your goal.

For ladies, it is suggested that they observe any changes, especially while menstruating, carefully. Many might confuse the regular inflammation and abdominal pain during menstrual cycle to be an outcome or symptom of the diet otherwise.

What is the Metabolism Plan?

The metabolism plan isn't another faddy diet. It's a way of life. The human body works hard to process nutrients present in the food that we eat and then converts it to create energy, which the body needs to carry out daily functions and for the growth of the body. Metabolism is the process of keeping body cells healthy and working.

In most cases, poor metabolism leads to weight-gain. As a result, many people have problems with weight control. It is a matter of concern, as it is overtaking smoking as the leading cause of preventable deaths in the United States. Europe as well isn't far behind in the statistic, either.

When looking at that, it can all seem pretty grim, right? This leads to people believing in any diet plan that they can get their hands on, irrespective of its credibility or success. Many people on diets say they "can't eat that" or "that's not part of what I'm allowed," and eventually end up not being able to enjoy regular things like eating out with friends, or grabbing a quick lunch on the go. Some end up falling off the wagon completely.

The metabolism plan reduces inflammation, which is a cause of premature aging, weight gain, skin problems like eczema, autoimmune diseases like crowns disease and lupus. It even improves your thyroid function and hormonal balance.

The metabolism plan differs drastically from the fasting, military diets, all-out ban diets; because it banishes absolutely no food. It raises your body's metabolic rate using the food you are eating, by incorporating regular exercise into your life. That means, if you want that piece of chocolate, you can have it. Of course, overindulgence won't produce results, but by sticking to the metabolism plan, you will lose weight.

Devised by Lyn-Genet Recitas, an extremely capable dietitian whose "no-nonsense" approach to health has changed the mantra we've heard for 20 years. Earlier, the idea was to watch your calories and cut down the intake, which eventually led to weight loss. The moment you went back to old ways; you'd end up gaining back all the lost weight. This proves that counting calories and cutting down are a quick fix. It is not a permanent one, probably not a healthy one. The metabolism diet, on the other hand, takes a holistic approach and doesn't rely solely on food. It also makes into account blood type, age, sleeping pattern, physical activity, autoimmunity, etc. It is like looking at the bigger picture instead of fixing the body in bits and pieces which most of the diets out there, do. This food aims to bring the metabolism level back to where it should be; functioning correctly and improved health.

Debunking some misconceptions about metabolism

Many people believe that like their eye color they are born with a specific metabolism, which can't be changed. How many times have you seen a friend complain, "I have poor metabolism, that's why I can't lose weight?" That's not entirely true. Your metabolism is a direct result of what you eat, do and even your sleeping patterns. Yes, it takes time to change it and effort to, but unlocking the secret is not opening Pandora's Box or reinventing the wheel.

Metabolism is not the same person to person; Bad lifestyle choices, crash dieting, fasting, all lead to serious metabolic problems, which is why the metabolic diet differs from person to person. Some success stories revealed that people had been eating too little, and exercising too much. The metabolic plan cracks the code of your metabolism by taking your lifestyle into considerations; the kind of things that you can do within the constrictions of your daily routine. It also tries to uncover things that you are doing wrong that is secretly sabotaging your efforts. It brings so much clarity about how you can implement changes that will help you feel rested and energized, and also satisfied with the food you eat.

Understanding How Metabolism Works

Metabolism is a relatively commonly used word, but a pretty understood concept. Metabolism is the culmination of several different elements in the creation and destruction of protoplasm. Sounds complicated? It is, but you don't need to worry about that.

It is merely a series of chemical processes where cells produce heat & energy using the nutrients from food. This energy is then used to build compounds to carry out essential life functions like blinking, breathing, etc. The energy produced during metabolism also helps in the building of complex compounds like proteins, which are necessary for the growth and repair of tissues. People who exercise on a regular basis have increased metabolism. They weren't born with fast metabolism's, but they created one.

Why This Plan Works and Diets Don't!

Like we stated before, there are 9 billion people in the world, and not even two are the same. So why should one diet work for everyone? The Metabolism rate is unique, personal to you. Who said that chocolate and red wine were going to ruin your diet? The Metabolism diet doesn't keep you from enjoying your favourite meals. Instead, it focuses on moderation and physical activity.

The metabolism diet is devised by Lyn-Genet Recitas, who has taken a chemical formula for changing your metabolism and adapted it for each person, depending on their blood type, weight, age, and ailments. To fully take this diet onboard and run with it, you need to change your way of thinking. Like we stated before, metabolism doesn't just affect weight, it also affects nearly every part of your body, from premature aging to mood swings. After seeing how important your metabolism is and how understanding your body's unique genetic chemistry can affect your ability to eat better, live better and feel better.

How many diets did you start and then quit because they didn't produce the right results? More than a few, I'm sure. Most of the times after these diets, you feel miserable, depleted and defeated and you shouldn't have to. You didn't fail at the diet; the diet failed with you!

Chapter 2: Ways To Lose Weight Without Disturbing Your Personal Life Or Happiness Distressing

Step 1 – Time Yourself (have a time plan) When Eating Meals by Placing a Timer

Having enough time for meals is essential. The recommended duration for having meals is 20 to 30 minutes. The reason why this amount time is suggested is that individual often takes their meals because of a psychological hunger. In the subsequent paragraph, a further explanation is given.

As referred to in the previous paragraph, usually, food that is hastily taken is not properly digested. Moreover, an individual who hurriedly takes his meals is not emotionally satisfied because he didn't sit down to relax before or during meal time. Usually, the brain is supposed to tell the body when it is satisfying, but in a case of a quick mealtime, such a communication might not be well conveyed leading to an individual to feel unsatisfied shortly after taking meals.

Step 2 – Tell Someone Who's Close to You That You Are Watching What You Eat

Tell your friend, or partner or a colleague that you are watching what you're eating. This will give you extra motivation in their presence because you will always be reminded of the commitment you made and they will encourage you to keep going.

Step 3 – Create A Massive Batch of Green Tea and Freeze It

You may not be able to drink hot green tea when you are in a hurry. However, you may want to make a pitcher of the green tea in your home and store it in your freezer during the night. The amazing benefits of green tea are that it is rich in antioxidants among other nutrients that will aid in your weight loss and appetite suppression.

Step 4- If You Mess Up and Fall Off the Wagon, Get Back On

There's no point in starting the metabolism diet if you are not determined to reach the goal. Try not to stock your refrigerator, if that is what it takes, for you to not eat the wrong foods at the wrong time. Analyze the behavior and the mistakes you made in the past and regularly tell yourself, "I'm not doing that again."

Step 5: Turn Off Your Phone, Tablet, And All Artificial Lights 2 Hours Before Bed.

As referred to earlier, light determines the metabolism and also the amount of sleep that our bodies get. For our bodies to stay healthy and cut weight, we require a rest of 7-8 hours but the electrical appliances ought to be switched off. Failure to turn off such devices would mean the brain is not given time to relax and consequently lead to inadequate sleep, overeating during the day and reduced metabolism.

Chapter 3: Key Commandments To Unlock Your Perfect Metabolism

Fix Your Sugar

Did you know that sugar is one of the most addictive substances in the world and that people experience withdrawal, cravings when trying to stop? The urge to eat vast amounts of sugar is not unheard. However, sugar is the direct cause of many health ailments, for example, Candida.

Candida is a type of yeast infection, which can affect anyone. Most people, who have it, don't even know that they have it and have had it for years. Once a person stops their intake of sugar, the candida (which causes problems in the skin, weight, digestive disorders and brain fog) die off, and the person feels much better. It takes a few weeks, but it does happen.

The Importance of Fats

All fats aren't created equally, of course. Yes, there are good fats. However, think if it's worthwhile to continue to eat it on a regular basis. For example, the metabolism diet relies heavily on Omega 3 and healthy fats, which are found in oily fish, like salmon.

Have you ever drained a pan after you have fried a steak and let the fat solidify? If you have you all know what it is, and it's truly disgusting. Could you imagine drinking that, eating it? No. However, people fail to remember that it happens when they consistently eat animal fats, saturated fats like butter and creams. Healthy fats that originate from nuts, oily fish and seeds are the kind of fats you do want in your life.

Heal Your Gut

Crohn's diseases, colitis, Irritable Bowel Syndrome are a few examples of disorders caused by an unhealthy gut. These are being diagnosed at an epidemic rate. People affected by these diseases have an enormous impact on their life, and these conditions come with an enormous societal cost. It becomes difficult to enjoy a healthy life.

So naturally, it is of utmost importance that we start the healing process here. First, we need to understand the problem area, which is, our entire digestive system. Digestion begins from the mouth, followed by the esophagus, the stomach, the small intestine, the large intestine, the rectum and ends at the anus. The tube is connecting all these organs from where the food passes called the GI tract or the gastrointestinal tract.

The good news is that we can heal the gut by taking easy steps and making a few changes as listed below:

- **Get rid of inflammatory foods and toxins:** We recommend losing processed food, GMO, grains, gluten, sugar and dairy from your diet.

- **Reduce stress:** It gets difficult to be stress-free in our fast-paced lives. We recommend taking small walks, practicing yoga, getting adequate sleep or meditating to name a few.

- **Rebalance Gut bacteria:** Include probiotics and probiotic-rich food foods to your diet. To name a few: Raw Cheese, Brine-cured olives, Apple cider vinegar, Coconut yogurt, Fermented vegetables like gherkin pickles, kimchi, etc.

Food Intolerances

Most people aren't even aware that they have food intolerances until the pain and adverse effects become intolerable. The most common food intolerances are gluten, dairy and animal products. Continuing to eat food that we are intolerant to make you extremely sick, bloated and ill in the long term. A very high priority of the metabolism diet is that it will keep you from eating food that your body doesn't want you to eat.

Losing the Harmful Weight

Besides being unsightly and embarrassing, excessive weight is overtaking Smoking as the Leading cause of preventable death in the US. That number I expected to rise. This generation is set to be the first one on record who will live less time than their parents.

Diabetes is now being diagnosed in children as young as 5. Type 2 Diabetes is entirely preventable and a direct result of obesity. A person with Type 2 Diabetes will live on average 25 years than a person who does not have it, and their quality of life will be severely compromised as a result.

Yes, it's fun to eat, and yes, unhealthy food often tastes good, but in the end; it's not worth it. For the sake of holding yourself back and staying on your mission, you could be forfeiting quite a lot.

Furthermore, obesity is directly linked to depression. Meaning, it affects every facet of your life. Your body, your mind and also your wellbeing are torn to pieces. People who suffer from obesity are also more likely to commit suicide, and all obese people have a shorter lifespan than their regular weight counterparts.

Lowering Inflammation

Inflammation is something that's caused a few things; diet and hormones. Inflammation of the gut leads to water retention and means that we suffer from bloat. This can be extremely uncomfortable and can often compromise your quality of life.

A simple way to reduce inflammation is to understand, using the metabolic diet, what is causing the inflammation and to stay away from it. It's pretty simple when you put into these constraints.

Poor Sleep, Stress and A Life Spent On a Tablet or Phone

Light plays an essential part in our bodies sleep, and metabolism signals and one of the most critical parts of our lives is sleeping. To successfully lead a healthier life and lose weight, we must sleep 7-8 hours a day. Some of the things that prevent us from sleeping are gadgets that cause overstimulation to our senses and lead us not to have enough sleep; which, in turn, leads to us eating more during the day and our metabolism functioning at a slower rate.

The Importance of Nutrients

Most people don't even know what nutrients are, never mind if they are deficient in them. When your body is depleted of nutrients and electrolytes, then it doesn't function. Your metabolism doesn't work correctly because your cells can't be repaired, they are too busy trying to compensate for all the damage you are doing to yourself by being depleted in necessary nutrients like potassium, vitamin D; which are all very essential to our body.

Water, Water, Water

Staying hydrated is the best gift you can give to your body. Not only does it keep the intestines flexible and smooth but also allows a natural movement of food all the through the GI tract. The Institute of Medicine recommends drinking 9 cups (2.2. liters) of water for women and 13 cups (3 liters) for men daily.

In the midst of our busy schedules, we often forget to drink water. You can change that by carrying a water bottle around, drinking water before every meal, drinking after exercising, etc. You can also eat your water by consuming foods with higher water content. E.g., Cucumbers, Zucchinis, Tomatoes, Pineapple, Watermelon, Strawberries, etc.

Brush Your Teeth After Meals!

Brushing your teeth after meals and using mouthwash will help prevent you from reaching for snacks in between meals (especially after your main evening meal), properly brushing your teeth will leave the minty taste in your mouth and you won't want to grab a bag of potato chips after your dinner.

Exercising More Efficiently

Don't s set unrealistic goals for yourself like a 4-hour workout every day, start off slowly. Find things which fit into your schedule as a worker, mom, wife. Try even just walking to work or getting off the bus a few stops early.

If you set yourself an unattainable goal then you will break it, and then you might adopt the famous mantra; "ok, I messed up on my diet I might as well forget everything." This is a dangerous way of thinking and believes me, it won't get you very far, and you all feel like a constant failure. Download a fitness app to monitor how many steps you are taking a day, many Americans only walk as many as 1000 steps a day, trying upping that to 4000 and you will see results long term.

The metabolism diet also stresses that what worked for someone else, might not work for you, so your exercise, like diet has to be tailored to your needs, your body and your capabilities as a person.

Chapter 4: Simple Detox Guides

Importance of Detoxification

Detox is a word that is thrown around a lot. Detox teas, Detox Retreats, etc. But what does it mean? It is a process of getting rid of toxic or unhealthy substances (read: foods and habits as well). In the process, you try and abstain from anything that enhances the buildup of toxins in the body.

The purpose is to help the digestive organs to metabolize and flush toxins out of our system. This can be done by lowering the toxins that we unnecessarily put in our bodies on a daily basis and by including nutrients that are required for the proper functioning of the body.

How to tell if my body needs to Detox?

There's no test to see if you need to detox. Take a look at all the symptoms below. If you have more than 4 of these, your body needs to detox.

- White bacteria coated tongue and foul breath

- Retention of fluids in the body/or congested sinuses
- Increased belly or visceral fat
- Regular unhealthy cravings and issues related to blood sugar
- Problematic Gallbladder and absence of gallbladder (if you have had it removed)
- Bloating in the abdomen
- Excessive sweating/ heating of the body
- Resistance to weight loss
- Acne, rosacea, itchy skin
- Waking up tired post adequate sleep
- Frequent mood swings
- Autoimmune diseases
- Multiple Chemical sensitivity aka Idiopathic Environmental Intolerances (I.E.I) – getting lightheaded from drinking alcohol or getting anxious from smelling fragrances.

- Insomnia or/and easily awakened around 1-4 a.m.

Guide and Charts to Help You Detox the Right Way

Set a date when you will start your detox and monitor each day how you feel. Detoxing can be light, enjoyable even, and for some, it can result in headaches, mood swings, and digestive problems. Detoxing Is an incredibly personal experience, and it should be treated as such.

Making it personal

Not everyone wants to detox to reach a specific weight on the scale. Many just want to rid of illnesses which have plagued them for a long time, like skin conditions, depression, etc. Therefore, it's essential to make your detox personal to you and your needs.

A person who is satisfied with their weight but is suffering from chronic illness doesn't need to follow the same detox plan as someone with a BMI of 40. (BMI- Body Mass Index; it is your weight in kilograms over your height in meters squared). A BMI of 18.5-24.9 suggests normal weight. Anyone beyond 30 is obese.

Your age is also an important thing to take into consideration when thinking about detoxification. Age affects everything, especially our metabolism, and generation must be a very core factor when thinking about what approach to take to detox and which one is the most suited and relevant.

There are a lot of detox plans available today, and each targets a particular problem area. We will not discuss each at length, but there are a few simple ways that can help you detox at home and make it a part of your lifestyle.

- **Drink Green Tea:** Due to the antioxidants present in green tea, it not only helps in burning fat but also in boosting the immune system. It improves the metabolic rate and flushes out toxins from the body.

- **Eat Raw vegetables:** A few vegetables contain sulfur, which naturally helps the liver to push out toxins. These are cabbage, kale, carrots, broccoli, beets, Brussels sprouts to name a few. If you don't enjoy eating them raw, you can also juice them or add them to smoothies.

- **Include Omega 3 rich foods:** Omega 3 fatty foods help in lubricating the intestinal wall and contain fatty acids, which aid in the proper functioning of the liver. This helps the body in eliminating toxins from the body. Some examples are; avocado oil, walnut oil, fish oil. Olive oil, flax seed oil.

- **Avoid Starch and Sugar in your diet:** These foods lead to the building of toxins in the body. They cause a lot of illnesses and poorly affect the immunity of the body. You should avoid foods rich in carbohydrates like potatoes, pumpkins, yams, sweet potatoes, corn, etc.

- **Exercise:** This not only helps in keeping the heart and lungs healthy but also helps in flushing out toxins from the body. The more you exercise, the more you feel the need to hydrate your body. The water intake helps the kidneys to function better and get rid of toxins quickly. Exercising helps in the proper functioning of the digestive system.

Chapter 5: Eat And Cleanse At The Same Time.

Importance of incorporating the right foods into your plan

The foods to avoid and include mentioned in chapter 4 are a quick-acting way to kick-start the detox. We have consciously recommended foods that are easy to find and do not disappoint the taste buds either.

Delicious & Healthy fat-burning meals

Did you know that spice is one of the world's natural fat burners? Adding it to a simple, healthy dish not only makes it enjoyable to eat but also actually, helps to burn fat.

Here are some examples:

Broccoli and Eggs: This is a simple meal for breakfast which does not require much time to take but will keep your body healthy and satisfied. With just 30 calories per serving of broccoli, you are assured to be filled with fiber. The eggs, on the other hand, control your appetite to help stave off those unwanted cravings.

Add red pepper spice to anything! Do you remember that diet where everyone was drinking lemonade and cayenne pepper? Yes, it was stupid, but the cayenne pepper is a great fat burner. Adding Cayenne Pepper to a Salmon and vegetable dish will pack a punch and burn fat while totally satiating you.

When to eat to intensify detoxification?

Eating in the morning after you have exercised for 30 minutes is ideal. Waking up and drinking water, allowing your body to absorb that for some time and then starting the day with a detoxifying smoothie is what you need to get things "going" in the morning.

Eating a late dinner is not a good idea. Like we mentioned before, adequate sleep is essential for the body to stay stress-free. Not only does eating late cause disrupted sleep, but also gives wrong signals to the body. Eating heavy meals late at night makes the organization believe that a shortage of food is expected and hence it starts to store fat. This body tries to work hard to digest food as a result of which sleep is affected. The body doesn't get adequate rest, making us emotionally unstable the next day which leads to unhealthy cravings and so on. It's a cycle, and so we need to start at the first step. Dinner should always be 2-3 hours before bedtime or before you start settling down for the night.

Chapter 6: 10 Minutes' Alternative Workout. Two Weeks Plan And What To Eat.

What Should Your Shopping List Look?

Your shopping list should have spices, basil, cinnamon (very important for reducing inflammation), vegetables, leafy greens, nuts (all kinds), salmon, sardines, coconut oil, etc.

10-Minute Fat Burning Exercises Plan and 2-Weeks Diet Plan

While we understand that all bodies are different and everyone has a different rate of metabolism, we have come up with exercise plans that will suit all. The idea is to incorporate these into your daily workout. Some of you might be happy with your body after working out only for a couple of minutes while some of you might not be satisfied even after long hours of workout. The idea behind this workout plan is to get you started. You can gradually and eventually alter the time according to how your body responds to the workout. We recommend adding an extra 2-5 minutes slowly to the workout every week. This will not only help you increase your strength but also assist in bettering your metabolism. We suggest that you don't stop exercising altogether at any point. Exercising relieves stress, and lessens the burden, the easier it is to keep those extra pounds away.

Here are a few tips for 10-minute exercise plan:

Squat-Thrust Push-Up

Melting excess calories can be as fast as trying out some cardio routines. Try out Keli Roberts' (*10-Minute Cardio Kick Box* creator) pumped up cardio workout. Within 10 minutes, you will have burnt 150 calories.

Skipping Rope

Duration: approximately two minutes.

Start by jumping twice per turn; ensure to land on balls of feet softly.

Squat-Thrust Push-Up

Duration: between second to the third minute. Stand with your arms by their side and feet apart. Squat and bring your hands to the floor beside your feet. With legs in a plank pose, jump. Hop with your feet towards the inside of hands. Hop, while reaching for the ceiling with your fingertips and repeat the process.

Side-Plank Squat-Thrust Push-Up

Skipping Rope

Duration: between third to fourth minutes.

Jump once per turn.

Side-Plank Squat-Thrust Push-Up

Duration: Lasts between minute four to five.

Repeat minute two to three. However, after completion of push-up, move your body weight onto your right hand and outer right foot. Rotate your body towards the right and extend your left arm upwards perpendicularly while keeping hips raised. Turn back to the middle and repeat the routine for the left side. To start, hop your feet back and jump up. Repeat the method.

Squat-Thrust Push-Up with Leg Lifts

Skipping Rope

Duration: between minute five to six.

Jump once per turn.

Squat-Thrust Push-Up with Leg Lifts

Duration: between minute six to seven.

Repeat minute two to three. When push-up is complete, lift left leg about a foot. Lower left leg and repeat with the right. Jump up. Repeat routine.

Squat-Thrust Push-Up with Mountain Climbers

Skipping Rope

Duration: between minute seven to eight.

Jump once per turn.

Squat-Thrust Push-Up with Mountain Climbers

Duration: between minute eight to nine.

Repeat minute two to three. When you complete the push-up, hop your right foot beneath your hips to the floor then bounce the foot back, stretching the leg behind you. Bring left foot forward. While alternating sides, complete 5 hops on each leg. Jump up. Repeat routine.

Skipping Rope

Duration: Minute nine to ten.

Jump once per turn.

Here Are a Few Tips to Burn Fat While Toning and Defining Your Abs and Core

This ten-minute workout not only helps in toning but it goes beyond to help in losing belly fat, defining abdominals and strengthening of the core. Doing core exercises in high-intensity intervals will give you perfect abs in no time. Prepare yourself to burn that abs. Expect good results and modify your lifestyle with the way you eat, look and feel.

Equipment You Need: Yoga mat and A Record Timer

What to Do: For 25 seconds, do the exercise and rest for twelve seconds every after completing a circuit. For best results, repeat this work out thrice a week. You may want to search for videos on the net to know the appropriate way of working out.

Challenge: Performing the Fat Burning Workout while doing the metabolism plan

Complete 1 round of circuits 1 – 5

Circuit One: Perform Plank Jacks

Circuit Two: Perform Plank Jacks and Toe Touches.

Circuit Three: Perform Plank Jacks, Toe Touches, and Plank Jacks

Circuit Four: Perform Plank Jacks, Toe Touches, Plank Jumps again then do the Workout for Lower Belly and Hip Lift.

Circuit Five: Repeat Circuit 4 and add Jumping Squat Thrust at the end.

Why is it okay to start with 10-minute workouts?

Contrary to common belief, these 10-minute workouts, actually work and give desired results. We suggest you do it in the morning for best results. Let us explain a little about how and why these workouts are better than no exercise or longer workouts.

Doable

These are easy to say yes. The mental block that keeps you from working out or joining that aerobics class or the early morning run that you keep procrastinating about is removed. You find fewer excuses to dismiss a 10-minute workout, so it is a perfect way to kick-start for beginners. For people with busy schedules, these 10-minute workouts seem manageable.

Gets you committed to the goal

Once you are comfortable with the routine, you start realizing how good you feel about exercising. It is no more an extra activity. It becomes a part of your lifestyle, and you don't shy away from putting in additional efforts. Some of you might end up adding a couple of more minutes to the workout while a few of you might finally go for that early morning run or doing any other physical activity that catches your fancy.

These workouts are just as effective

The short exercises are better because they keep you focused as compared to a more extended workout where you're just sloppy and looking for breaks. We recommend mornings as the perfect time to do these exercises because they leave you feeling refreshed and energized which gives a higher chance for you to make better choices during the day.

Improved consistency

The most important factor determining the success of any workout plan is consistency. We all start motivated, and as days go by and the excitement dies, we come up with excuses and go back to old ways. With 10-minute workouts, it is difficult to come with excuses and dismiss it quickly. Everyone has that kind of time in their day to work towards a healthy body and mind. It is more efficient than long hours of working out that only happen a few times a months because it is easier to work out every day for 10 minutes.

What we truly need is effective weight loss that is also sustainable. This is not for a week or a month; this is a lifestyle change which, if followed correctly, will keep away any desire to revert to old ways.

Chapter 7: How Will I Know If Things Are Working?

What Should You Expect?

The answer is pretty simple; during detoxing you feel dilapidated, unwell and typically tired, with a weak mood, headache, and some brain fog. This will peak at around 10-14 days and then will go down over time. This is, of course, dependent on how many toxins you had in your body, how old you are and how your metabolism and general health is as a whole, there is no one answer to this question. However, with time, you will learn better your body signs, when to push a detox further and when to take a break.

Truth About Detoxing

There is no one size fits all approach to this, if so, there would be no obesity in the world. Your body will do the talking, and you will have to listen to its nuances, ways and cooperate with it. Detoxing isn't forever, it's something that lasts a few months, and then you can start to live a clean, healthy and long life. Detoxing is not something which has to take over your life entirely. However, it's suggested to take some time off work or school so that you can dedicate your time to recovery, and not be distracted by other things.

Chapter 8: How Your Body Answers, What Does It Want, What Should You Do, Regularly.

Tips for Long-Term Weight Loss Success

Losing weight is not a particularly difficult process to undertake. If you are looking to slim into a dress, then eating nothing but boiled cabbage for one week will produce some good results. That's why the covers of all the glossy magazines boast "Lose 10lbs in one week" and "Beyoncé's 20lb weight loss ahead of her performance in dream girls". This is entirely possible; there is no hard science in starving the body of nutrients and creating a deficit. The only problem is that the pendulum which swings in the direction of weight loss will quickly turn back; leaving the person who lost the weight with more weight than they started and start a cycle of yo-yo dieting, which is a cycle many people are stuck.

Losing a few pounds in a week, or even a few days, is entirely achievable, one merely needs to put far less into their body, suffer acute hunger and excerpt an abnormal amount of exercise. This isn't healthy.

Long-term weight loss comes when people take a look at themselves seriously, see what their actual capabilities and capacities are; what they can do and what they are not able to do. An unachievable prerequisite in a diet, for example, walking 20km per day and cutting out a food type which you rely heavily on upon.

Weight loss is just the start of the entire journey; you can think of it, I suppose as the birth of the person, and then the rest of the ride is them growing up, learning, changing, altering and moving forward and away from the mistakes they have made in the past. In all trueness, weight was never gained overnight, or by a week of overindulgence. It creeps on over time. Yes, of course, there are some health factors can, of course, affect the weight of an individual but this is rarely the reason people are overweight.

After much study, scientist felt like they might have found the "fat gene," but they did not. It's true that obesity runs in families, but it's a natural assumption to say that the behavior which the parent learned from their parent, passed it down to the child and the cycle of obesity continues.

Obesity is said to be a crisis of our generation, who are expected to live less than their parents, which is the first time in history which this has happened. We don't have the facilities to deal with this and address this. Obesity-related illnesses cost every government millions or billions of dollars per year in care. Preventative care and knowledge have not been the attitude which has been adopted. This means that it is up to the individual themselves to make sure their weight loss is long term and that they don't need to result in yo-yo dieting and ruining their metabolism and body irrevocably.

Here's Some Go- Tips for Long-Term Weight Loss

Broaden your taste buds.

Each time you go to the supermarket, buy something you wouldn't ordinarily purchase and try it. Adding new healthy foods to your diet will mean you will have healthier choices to make when eating on the go and also eating out with friends. Furthermore, you will spend less time in the Supermarket eventually, so you will have a succinct list of items you wish to purchase.

Never go shopping on an empty stomach.

Going shopping on an empty stomach is like finding the water fountain in the middle of the desert. You are going to make poor choices and snack while shopping. Instead, create a list on your phone, listen to your favourite podcast and walk around while carefully and mindfully making your purchases, instead of loading your cart with calorie dense, nutritionally deficit "quick fix "food, which will answer your hunger pangs immediately.

Taking this idea to another level is not going to a supermarket at all.

Do all your grocery shopping online. This is the only way you can guarantee to never stray from your list, snack while you are on the go or be tempted by product placement. Your pocket and your waistline will thank you. By grocery shopping online you are changing your entire attitude towards how you look at food. Food is there to be enjoyed, food is also something to be experienced in a social context, but the food is ultimately fuel. By changing your approach to food, you will see that, like you wouldn't put diesel in your petrol car, you can't put trash in your body.

How Often Should I Detox?

This is an incredibly unique question, and it depends entirely on you. Usual signs of needing to detox are seeing symptoms of chronic illnesses returning, candida and also a brain fog feeling, accompanied by digestive issues such as constipation. Once you have done one or two detoxes, you will feel yourself when you need to do your next. Detoxing doesn't need to be something which you run from and dread, often it's just part of your routine, like clearing out the cupboards in the kitchen every few months.

Constipation and getting back up is one of the classic signs that you may need to detox and also skin problems, like acne or psoriasis getting worse or returning. Often when we need to do a detox, we know that it is something which needs to happen. We start to feel sluggish, old symptoms begin to return, and your body feels it's due for its regular "reset." This doesn't need to be a time to dread; one must always remember the incredible feeling one feels after a detox; clean, cleared and free minded!

Do I Need to Give Up My Favourite Food, Alcohol, Coffee, Fast Foods?

This varies from person to person. The entire approach to the metabolism diet is taking each person and their unique self into consideration. Alcohol is severely detrimental to weight loss and stopping drinking alcohol has terrific benefits for your living. Furthermore, alcohol causes inflammation; when your body absorbs alcohol, it swells up and retains more water, making it quite uncomfortable the day after a night on the town. Binge Drinking is terrible in many ways; not only does it cause severe damage to the liver but it also lowers temptations to eat irresponsibly.

Alcohol dehydrates the body, regardless of what drink it is causing an insatiable appetite and thirst. Heavy alcohol consumption does not have a place in a detox diet as it is impossible for the liver to fully recover and cleanse, while it's trying to break down the alcohol. The liver is a very resilient organ, so it does metabolize alcohol well, however, taking a break from drinking does the liver a world of good. If you do decide to have one or two drinks, make sure that you flush your liver system out with a lemon water cleanse the next day. This is the best way to expedite cleansing of the liver.

When asked if you need to give up your favourite food to detox the answer is; it depends on what your favourite food is. If your favourite food is something which your body cannot metabolize and causes you chronic issues- the sensible and kind thing to do to yourself would forgo it.

Coffee is another one that most people find very hard. Coffee is another drink which dehydrates us and is highly addictive. People who are giving up coffee experience tension headaches, extreme fatigue, mood swings, confusion; symptoms which are seen when patients give up a lifetime of drug and alcohol choices. Coffee is healthy in moderation, and for the metabolism, diet detox is not required.

When asked if giving up fast food is necessary, I do want to ask; what is fast food? Fast food is a Frankenstein product which has been created in a factory similar to your phone which you hold in your hand, assembled in an assembly line similar to that of your clothes, shipped, packaged and sent to a franchise near you. The list of ingredients in fast food is incomprehensible to most chefs. Yes, people are more aware now, and they know that items such as "high fructose" corn syrup is wrong, but that's just one component of fast food.

Fast food relies heavily on the use of cheap, reusable fats for frying their burgers, chicken, and fries. This oil is always the most inexpensive oil which can be found on the market and is utilized at a level which the body is not used to digesting. Many people believe that fast food is just a way of life. Fast lives, fast cars, quick decisions, fast food. It doesn't need to be that way. Fast food is changing, with healthy salad bars continually opening, which offer variety, tasty and healthy alternatives to fried nuggets and chips. Fast food in the traditional sense does not even satisfy you for more than an hour or so, leaving you craving more after just a short period. By switching from fast food for your lunchtime work meal, to a home cooked meal or something from the salad bar, you are saving thousands of dollars in cash and pounds off of your waistline.

Will I Lose Weight During the Detox?

That depends on what the goal of the detox was and what your diet was like before the detox. If your diet was a short stack for breakfast, McMuffin and a snack and then pizza for dinner then yes, of course, you will lose weight on a detox diet because you will be cutting out an enormous portion of your daily fat intake immediately.

If, however, your diet was pretty good, but you wanted to address a specific health issue, such as a yeast infection, you may not experience any weight loss, but you will experience some effects of the toxins "die off."

Challenges to Expect-If Any

Feeling sluggish

Toxins are the fuel which your body is using to keep itself going when you are on a detox diet so imagine it as low-quality gasoline. Your body will feel sluggish; you may have a strange coat on your tongue as your body is trying to purge the toxins out. It's challenging to be restricting and changing your diet and all the more while having bad physical feelings from it. It's hard to adhere to a detox when it seems your body is telling you to stop. However, this isn't the case; the case is that your body has been storing up all these toxins for so long that the final release of them is difficult for your body to go through. A good detox can sync you back into rhythm with your body, in a way you never were before.

Skin changes

Your skin, the most prominent organ in your body will go through a severe change, and it's important to scrub your skin to get the blood flow going and the toxins out or even lie in a bath of Epsom salts, which quite literally pull toxins out from inside of your body. Also just putting your feet in a bath of Epsom salts will produce some fantastic results and you will feel much better about it.

Mood changes

It is, of course, reasonable to experience tiredness, sluggishness, changes of mood (not dissimilar to the differences found when women are going through their monthly cycles). The worse the junk is that you were putting in your body, the more aggressive the detox is going to be. If you were heavily reliant on junk-food alcohol, complex carbohydrates then you can expect to have quite a severe reaction; headaches, sleepiness, fogginess, loose bowel movements and an inability to wake up in the morning. Bad breath is also a side effect which can be managed by gargling coconut oil which helps to draw the toxins out from inside your mouth.

A detox is never fun to experience, but the effects can indeed be reduced by resting, drinking plenty of water, scrubbing your body, sitting in Epsom salt baths and taking several deep breaths. No one can go through the detox for you, just like no one can go through childbirth for you. It's something you need to go through on your own, and it will be personal. You will know when the detox is at its peak and when things are starting to clear out; the moments of clarity and the well-being we feel as we begin to feel better is the prize for these efforts.

Chapter 9: Stable Metabolism Through Alternative Great/Easy/Fun Life Aspects.

Enjoyable Ways to Boost Metabolism in Achieving Homeostasis On Body Weight Regulation

Dimming lights and wearing an earmark

There are many ways to enjoy boosting your metabolism. Let's start with the one that requires no effort; sleeping. Your metabolic rate is raised from the deep REM state of sleep, so keeping the lights in your room as low as possible is a fantastic start. Wearing an earmark is also highly recommended if you need to block out any streetlamp or any artificial light from outside.

(REM or rapid eye movement sleep is a phase of sleep with rapid movement of eyes, while the body is getting into the resting stage).

Setting your daily targets

Every phone has a pedometer now, so it's easy to keep track of your physical activity regarding walking. Setting yourself a goal of 3 miles a day for starters is pretty conservative. That's just 45 minutes at a brisk pace around the neighbourhood listening to your favourite podcast. Do not waste this time by catching up on work-related emails- it's essential to have a separate time for personal and professional activities. This way, walking can be a real treat. Sometimes, when you are listening to your favourite podcasts one after the other and enjoying them, you will not even notice that you have walked more than your target for the day! We recommend gradually increasing the distance to about 6 miles in 90 minutes. The idea is to burn 500 calories or more every day. Because to lose 1 kg of weight in a week the body needs to burn 500 extra calories per day.

Doing exercise whenever you can

We are trying to bring about a lifestyle change and not just a quick fix for any of your problems. The idea is to bring about changes in your daily life, in activities that you do every day. At work, you can walk around after every 45 minutes. This keeps your muscles happy and also betters your metabolism. It prevents you from crunching your neck over the screen and leaving work feeling tired and not up for any healthy activity.

Life isn't all about counting calories. Whatever form of physical activity you like apart from the ones mentioned in the plan, add it to your routine. E.g., If, you enjoy going to the park with the kids, then don't sit and be on your phone while they play, instead use that time to walk laps around the playground or play with them if that is something that you enjoy.

If you like to shop then forget elevators, use the stairs, make a point of walking into every store in the mall, even if it's something which doesn't immediately sound like it will generate a lot of exercises; it actually will!

Bonus Chapter: 30-Day Metabolism Meal Plan Tips!

When you are feeling your lowest amount of exercise, eating junk day in, day out, it's hard to find the real motivation to get going, get ready and say "Ok, today is this day." Sure, it's hard to go through detox and live your life healthily, but it's just as hard to look in the mirror and not recognize who's even looking at you.

Every single long-term weight loss journey started off just like this, you need to see yourself at the finish line, having achieved your goals; slimmer, happier and functioning better than you ever imagined.

Let's Take a Look at The Typical 7 Day Meal Plan For Metabolism Diet:

Breakfast

Egg White Omelet

Ingredients

- 229 calories of spinach
- chopped onion and tomatoes (mix half a cup)
- whole egg and half a cup liquid egg
- whites

Egg Avocado Toast

Ingredients

- 270 calories berries
- Tomato and parsley salad
- Diced cucumber
- ¼ avocado
- 1 hard-boiled eggs or poached egg
- 250 calories 1 hard-boiled eggs
- ¼ avocado spread on toast
- 1-piece whole-wheat toast

Cheese and Turkey Crackers

Ingredients

- Oats; 350 calories skim milk, 300 calories almond milk, Cinnamon, 4 walnuts and ½ a cup of oatmeal cooked in unsweetened almond milk with raisins

- Turkey breast; 2 cheese wedges, sliced cucumber, 260 calories for both spinach and fresh dill on whole-grain crisp crackers

French Pancakes

Ingredients

- 1 egg and 1 banana
- Spices
- ¼ Greek yogurt
- Cinnamon
- 300 calories 2 tbsp. slivered almonds

Procedure

- Mash and cook on a pan both the egg and banana and spray with cooking spray
- Add your favourite spices and put on top ¼ Greek yogurt, cinnamon and 2 tbsp. of 300 calories of slivered almonds

Green Yoghurt and Lemon

Ingredients

- 340 calories honey

- Apples

- Cherries

- Fresh Green Yoghurt

Lunch

Sandwich: Israeli Tahini and Turkey

Ingredients

- Whole-wheat bread-1
- 3 oz. turkey breast
- ½ sweet potatoes
- 365 calories Tahini mixed with salt and lemon

Procedure

- Microwave for 7 minutes 1 piece whole-bread and 3 oz. turkey breast together with ½ sweet potato
- Add 365 calories tahini that is mixed with salt and lemon

Hummus with fresh cut veggies

Ingredients

- Lemon and tahini
- Pepper
- Salt
- chickpeas
- Mushrooms
- Olive oil
- Peppers
- 1 broccoli
- Cauliflower
- 470 of any other veggies

Procedure

- Cut cauliflower one broccoli, peppers, and mushrooms
- Mix chickpeas with olive oil, salt, pepper, lemon and tahini and place in bowl

- Add 470 calories of any other veggies

Artichoke Pasta with Vegetables

Ingredients

- Wheat pasta

- Fresh spinach

- Dry white wine

Procedure

- Boil whole wheat pasta in a pot

- Add one cup of fresh spinach and some dry white wine

- Pour out over drained pasta and serve

Chicken and Salad (Avocado Cucumber)

Ingredients

- 400 calories lime juice
- Fresh cilantro
- ½ diced cucumber
- ½ diced avocado
- 2 tbsp. olive oil
- Chicken breast
- Pepper
- Salt

Spaghetti Squash, Chicken, Mushrooms and Spinach

Ingredients

- Spaghetti squash length
- Scoop out seeds
- Chicken
- Fresh spinach
- mushrooms

Procedure

- Cut a spaghetti squash in half length-wise and scoop out seeds, and after that place flesh-side down on a pan
- Cook in the oven for 45 minutes
- Take out the squash with a fork and place in a bowl.
- In a different pan wait until the chicken is brown and ready
- Wilt a little of fresh spinach

- add the chicken and mushrooms then serve

Stuffed Chicken Breasts (Almond and Artichoke) with crispy potato fries.

Ingredients

- Artichokes
- Spinach
- Almonds
- Parmesan
- Chicken breasts
- 1 Large sweet potato
- Cooking oil
- Dried basil
- tsp dried oregano
- salt
- 300 Calories pepper to taste.
- Can of tuna
- one minced green bell pepper,

- 2 minced scallions,
- 1/4 cup salsa,
- six pimento-stuffed olives,
- 309 calories Mayo (reduced Fat!!)

Procedure

- Mix the artichokes, spinach, almonds, Parmesan in a small bowl
- cooked the chicken breasts through for 5 to 7 minutes per side. Cook until it turns golden brown
- slice one large sweet potato into sticks and spray with cooking oil
- Mix with dried basil, tsp dried oregano, salt and 300 Calories pepper to taste.

Dinner

Smoked Salmon served with Baby Artichokes

Ingredients

- Salmon steak

- 433 calories Baby artichokes

Procedure

- Cook salmon steak at 375 degrees for close to 20 minutes

- Serve 433 calories baby artichokes

Fried Tuna Steak served with Vegetable Jumble
Ingredients

- 4-oz tuna steak

- 2tbsp olive oil

- 373 calories 1 serving the vegetable medley

Procedure

- Sear a 4-oz tuna steak in 2 tbsp. olive oil

- Serve with 1 serving vegetable medley 373 calories

Poached Bass with Capers, Parsley, and Fennel

Ingredients

- Fennel
- Parsley
- 350 calories Capers
- Procedure

Procedure

- Cook All the Fennel
- Mix Parsley and 350 calories Capers together in a Steamer

Pork Kebabs with Oregano

Ingredients

- Pork
- Veggies
- Vegetables
- Mushrooms
- Zucchini
- Wooden skewers
- 316 calories Stuff skewers

Procedure

- Take the fat off the Pork
- Put it in the microwave and Boil the Veggies and mix with vegetables if you like.
- soak wooden skewers in water
- Wash and cut vegetables into kebabs
- Stuff skewers, and Place on an indoor or outdoor grill and cook for 8 to 10 minutes.

Black Bean Chili and Corn

Ingredients

- Ground round beef
- 2tsp salt-free
- chili powder
- 14-ounces frozen corn
- Black bean
- 14-ounce can of fat-free
- Less sodium beef broth
- 1 15-ounce can of tomato sauce

Procedure:

- Mix ground round beef (1 lb.) with chili powder (2 tablespoons, salt-free)
- Blend the mixture in a huge Dutch oven
- Cook on medium-high heat for 6 minutes. Alternatively, until the beef browns.
- Constantly stir to crumble

- Drain the mixture and put back in the pan

- Stir in a bag containing a mixture of black bean and frozen corn (14-ounce) and one can of beef broth (less-sodium, fat-free, 14-ounce), and one can of tomato sauce (15-ounce)

- Boil

- Cover

- Reduce heat and allow it to simmer for 10 minutes

- Uncover and let it to simmer for 5 minutes while occasionally stirring

- Scoop chili into bowls

- If desired, put sour cream and onions topping on each serving.

  300 calories

Conclusion

This is just for you to get started. As you can see, with these meal options you are not going to be hungry. Furthermore, you are going to be addressing the problems that you have with food. When it's late at night and your sitting, not hungry with your hand in a bag of potato chips, you need to realize that it does not come from a place of hunger. It's vital to stop it; if not, it's possible to eat yourself to death emotionally.

Smoking is the number one cause of preventable death in the United States, overeating and obesity are overtaking. Which means, our children and children's children could potentially die younger than we do. Furthermore, they will suffer from a laundry list of health problems we do not, and levels of certain types of cancer will skyrocket to the point we may not be able to support them. The time has come and gone for us to teach healthy eating and habits in schools, we need to start from the womb and move forward.

No one needs to go far to see someone who is genuinely affected by obesity or by diseases caused by eating the wrong type of food consistently. This should be a thing of the past. We are well versed now, in the damages, which are caused by smoking, but when we sit around the dinner table and stuff ourselves with trans fats and feed our children the same, do we see the smoke we are blowing in their face or the cigarettes we are lighting to them?

This doesn't need to be the case; obesity is 100% preventable an 100% reversible. That's one of the reasons why it's such a lucrative business for those wanting to sell, get slim fast schemes or other scams. We've lived long enough to see fads come and go. However, nothing has addressed the issue in a big way. By understanding the metabolism, how it functions, how to control it, how to optimize it, we can start to scratch the surface of obesity and weight control. The future sometimes looks bleak, but a slight light has been shone, and there has come a time for us to accept the new ways and ideas, which are before us.

Obesity will continue to exist. However, we have a chance to decide, every one of us, if we want to be a statistic or not. We have the power, we know, we have the resources, metabolism isn't a mystery anymore, and neither is weight control. We have this covered.

Final Words

Thank you again for purchasing this book! I really hope this book is able to help you.

The next step is for you to **join our email newsletter** to receive updates on any upcoming new book releases or promotions. You can sign-up for free and as a bonus, you will also receive our "*7 Fitness Mistakes You Don't Know You're Making*" book! This bonus book breaks down many of the most common fitness mistakes and will demystify many of the complexities and science of getting into shape. Having all this fitness knowledge and science organized into an actionable step-by-step book will help you get started in the right direction in your fitness journey! To join our free email newsletter and grab your free book, please visit the link and signup: **www.hmwpublishing.com/gift**

Finally, if you enjoyed this book, then I would like to ask you for a favor, would you be kind enough to leave a review for this book? It would be greatly appreciated!

Thank you and good luck in your journey!

About the Co-Author

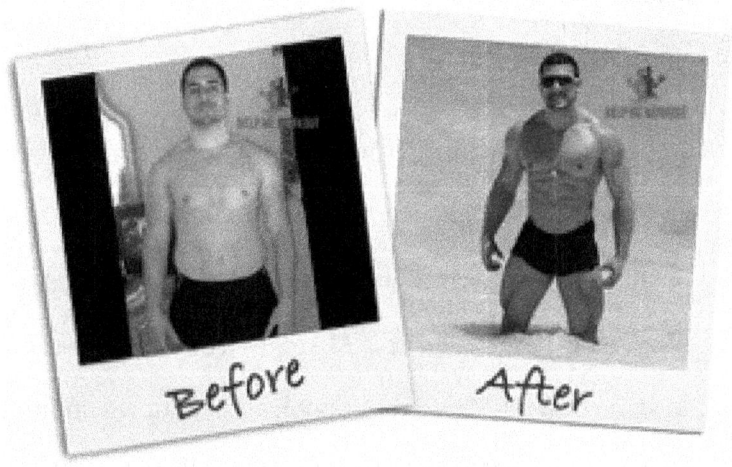

My name is George Kaplo; I'm a certified personal trainer from Montreal, Canada. I'll start off by saying I'm not the biggest guy you will ever meet and this has never really been my goal. In fact, I started working out to overcome my biggest insecurity when I was younger, which was my self-confidence. This was due to my height measuring only 5 foot 5 inches (168cm), it pushed me down to attempt anything I ever wanted to achieve in life. You may be going through some challenges right now, or you may simply want to get fit, and I can certainly relate.

For me personally, I was always kind of interested in the

health & fitness world and wanted to gain some muscle due to the numerous bullying in my teenage years about my height and my overweight body. I figured I couldn't do anything about my height, but I sure can do something about how my body looked like. This was the beginning of my transformation journey. I had no idea where to start, but I just got started. I felt worried and afraid at times that other people would make fun of me for doing the exercises the wrong way. I always wished I had a friend that was next to me who was knowledgeable enough to help me get started and "show me the ropes."

After a lot of work, studying and countless trial and errors. Some people began to notice how I was getting more fit and how I was starting to form a keen interest in the topic. This led many friends and new faces to come to me and ask me for fitness advice. At first, it seemed odd when people asked me to help them get in shape. But what kept me going is when they started to see changes in their own body and told me it's the first time that they saw real results! From there, more people kept coming to me, and it made me realize after so much reading and studying in this field that it did help me but it also allowed me to help others. I'm now a fully certified personal trainer and have trained numerous clients to date who have achieved amazing results.

Today, my brother Alex Kaplo (also a Certified Personal Trainer) and I own & operate this publishing venture, where we bring passionate and expert authors to write about health and fitness topics. We also run an online fitness website "HelpMeWorkout.com" and I would love to connect with by inviting you to visit the website on the following page and signing up to our e-mail newsletter (you will even get a free book).

Last but not least, if you are in the position I was once in and you want some guidance, don't hesitate and ask... I'll be there to help you out!

Your friend and coach,

George Kaplo
Certified Personal Trainer

Get another book for Free

I want to thank you for purchasing this book and offer you another book (just as long and valuable as this book), "Health & Fitness Mistakes You Don't Know You're Making", completely free.

Visit the link below to signup and receive it:

www.hmwpublishing.com/gift

In this book, I will break down the most common health & fitness mistakes, you are probably committing right now, and I will reveal how you can easily get in the best shape of your life!

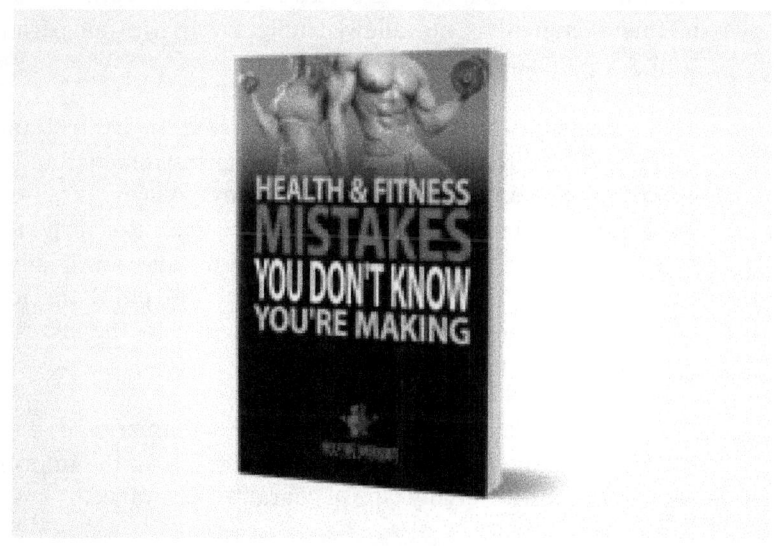

In addition to this valuable gift, you will also have an opportunity to get our new books for free, enter giveaways, and receive other valuable emails from me. Again, visit the link to sign up:

www.hmwpublishing.com/gift

Copyright 2017 by HMW Publishing - All Rights Reserved.

This document by HMW Publishing owned by the A&G Direct Inc company, is geared towards providing exact and reliable information in regards to the topic and issue covered. The publication is sold with the idea that the publisher is not required to render accounting, officially permitted, or otherwise, qualified services. If advice is necessary, legal or professional, a practiced individual in the profession should be ordered.

From a Declaration of Principles which was accepted and approved equally by a Committee of the American Bar Association and a Committee of Publishers and Associations.

In no way is it legal to reproduce, duplicate, or transmit any part of this document in either electronic means or in printed format. Recording of this publication is strictly prohibited, and any storage of this document is not allowed unless with written permission from the publisher. All rights reserved.

The information provided herein is stated to be truthful and consistent, in that any liability, in terms of inattention or otherwise, by any usage or abuse of any policies, processes, or directions contained within is the solitary and utter responsibility of the recipient reader. Under no circumstances will any legal responsibility or blame be held against the publisher for any reparation, damages, or monetary loss due to the information herein, either directly or indirectly.

The information herein is offered for informational purposes solely, and is universal as so. The presentation of the information is without contract or any type of guarantee assurance.

The trademarks that are used are without any consent, and the publication of the trademark is without permission or backing by the trademark owner. All trademarks and brands within this book are for clarifying purposes only and are the owned by the owners themselves, not affiliated with this document.

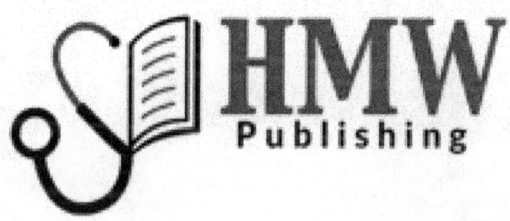

For more great books visit:

HMWPublishing.com

www.ingramcontent.com/pod-product-compliance
Lightning Source LLC
Chambersburg PA
CBHW071115030426
42336CB00013BA/2102